# HERBAL REMEDIES FOR PROSTATITIS

Empower Your Prostate Health With Herbs For Optimal Healing, Targeting Inflammation And Lasting Wellness

## DR. CARDEN KYRIE

# DISCLAIMER

The only goal of this book is informational. Every effort has been taken by the author and publisher to ensure that the information provided is accurate. But the material in this book is given "as is," without any express or implied representation, warranty, or condition as to its accuracy, completeness, or suitability for any particular purpose.

Any loss, damage, or injury resulting from using the information in this book, or from any action or decision made as a result of such use, will not be covered by the author's or publisher's liability. It is recommended that readers seek the assistance of a certified specialist for guidance specific to their situation.

The opinions and viewpoints conveyed in this book belong to the author and may not necessarily represent the official stance or policies of any specified organizations or people. Any likeness to real-life occurrences, places, or people—living or deceased—is wholly coincidental.

No specific product, service, or therapy discussed in this book is endorsed by the author or publisher. Any reference to goods or services is made only for informative reasons and is not intended as a recommendation or endorsement.

Before making any judgments or acting on any information, readers are urged to independently confirm it all. Any unfavorable effects or repercussions arising from the usage of the material included in this book are disclaimed by the author and publisher.

By using this book, you consent to absolving the publisher and author of any and all claims, obligations, or losses resulting from your use of the material in it.

I appreciate your cooperation and understanding.

# TABLE OF CONTENTS

# CHAPTER ONE

## INTRODUCTION TO PROSTATITIS
## RECOGNIZING PROSTATITIS

A considerable portion of men worldwide suffer from prostatitis, a complicated and sometimes misdiagnosed medical ailment marked by inflammation of the prostate gland. Producing seminal fluid, the prostate, a walnut-sized gland situated directly below the bladder, is essential to the male reproductive system. Acute bacterial infections and long-term nonbacterial inflammations are two different ways that prostatitis can present itself. The symptoms can have a major negative effect on a man's quality of life.

These symptoms may include pelvic pain or discomfort, trouble urinating, and sexual dysfunction. Because prostatitis can take many forms, it is crucial for those who want to take control of their health as well as medical professionals who want to treat patients well to understand the complexities of this condition.

# THE SIGNIFICANCE OF MALE HEALTH

Discussions about women's health have traditionally taken center stage when it comes to men's health, but in recent years, as societies have realized how important it is to address gender-specific health issues, men's health has gotten more attention. Men's health is more than just treating particular ailments; it's about being well generally, which includes mental, emotional, and physical components. Men have particular health problems, such as a greater incidence of heart disease, problems with their prostates, and a reluctance to seek medical attention. A healthier male population can be achieved through supporting proactive healthcare practices and increasing knowledge of these issues. Furthermore, a holistic approach to men's health recognizes the interdependence of several variables, such as genetics, environment, and lifestyle.

# THE FUNCTION OF HERBAL TREATMENTS

The use of herbal therapies has drawn attention to the quest for holistic health and well-being. For ages, people from many cultures have used herbal remedies, which are made from plants and other natural sources, because they may have medicinal effects. Herbal medicines have been investigated as supplemental or alternative treatments for illnesses like prostatitis in the context of men's health. Certain herbs are thought to have anti-inflammatory qualities, which may be especially helpful in reducing the inflammation brought on by prostatitis. Comprehending the function of herbal treatments entails taking into account their possible benefits, constraints, and the significance of evidence-based approaches. It takes a well-rounded strategy that incorporates both conventional medical knowledge and traditional wisdom to incorporate herbal treatments into men's healthcare.

Knowing the subtleties of prostatitis, appreciating the significance of men's health, and investigating the use of herbal medicines in medicine are related topics that add to a thorough knowledge of men's health. A more integrative and successful approach to men's health can be achieved by adopting a holistic viewpoint that incorporates traditional and herbal therapies alongside conventional medical procedures as societies change in how they approach healthcare.

# CHAPTER TWO

## SYNOPSIS OF PROSTATITIS

## TYPES AND DEFINITION OF PROSTATITIS

Inflammation of the prostate gland, a walnut-sized organ situated directly below the bladder in males, is the hallmark of the medical disorder prostatitis. Because it produces the seminal fluid that both nourishes and transports sperm, the prostate gland is an essential component of the male reproductive system. Based on its origin and clinical manifestation, prostatitis is a general word that encompasses a variety of illnesses affecting the prostate. It is further categorized into several kinds.

Acute bacterial prostatitis, chronic bacterial prostatitis, chronic prostatitis/chronic pelvic pain syndrome (CP/CPPS), and asymptomatic inflammatory prostatitis are the four main kinds of prostatitis. Caused by a bacterial infection, acute bacterial prostatitis is usually characterized by symptoms that appear suddenly, such as fever, chills, and difficulty urinating. Recurrent or persistent bacterial infections of the prostate are known as chronic bacterial prostatitis. The most prevalent type, known as CP/CPPS, is characterized by persistent pelvic discomfort and symptoms related to urination, whereas asymptomatic inflammatory prostatitis is discovered by chance when doing tests for other illnesses.

## TYPICAL SYMPTOMS

Depending on the type, pelvic pain or discomfort, lower back pain, painful and frequent urination, and sexual dysfunction are common symptoms of prostatitis. Fever and lethargy are other flu-like symptoms that some people may have, particularly in situations of acute bacterial prostatitis.

## REASONS AND DANGER ELEMENTS

There are many different reasons why prostatitis occurs, however, both acute and chronic bacterial prostatitis are frequently caused by bacterial infections.

Though the precise origin of CP/CPPS is yet unknown, a complicated interaction between variables like inflammation, an inflammatory reaction, and neuromuscular dysfunction is thought to be at play. A history of urinary tract infections, blockage of the bladder outlet, and recent urinary tract-related medical procedures are risk factors for prostatitis.

## CONVENTIONAL THERAPIES AND THEIR RESTRICTIONS

Alpha-blockers to relax the muscles in the bladder and prostate, anti-inflammatory drugs to reduce symptoms, and antibiotics to combat bacterial infections are common traditional therapies for prostatitis.

These methods are not without their drawbacks, though, particularly in CP/CPPS instances when the cause is unclear and antibiotic efficacy may be in doubt. Moreover, prolonged use of antibiotics may not treat the underlying causes of chronic prostatitis and may result in antibiotic resistance.

# USING HERBAL MEDICINE TO TREAT PROSTATITIS

The use of herbal medication is one of the alternative methods of managing prostatitis that has attracted increasing attention in recent years. Many people turn to herbal medicines because they may have anti-inflammatory and immune-modulating effects. The potential benefits of saw palmetto, quercetin, and rye grass pollen extract as herbal remedies for controlling symptoms of prostatitis are frequently studied. It's important to remember, though, that although some people find relief with herbal medicine, there is currently little scientific proof of their effectiveness. More research is required to determine their place in the treatment of prostatitis.

Prostatitis is a complex illness that comes in different forms, each with unique symptoms and difficulties.

# CHAPTER THREE

## RECOGNIZING THE HEALTH OF MEN

## FACTORS IMPACTING THE HEALTH OF MEN

Numerous factors, including both biological and environmental ones, have an impact on men's health. Genetics is a significant factor because people are predisposed to various health issues by birth. Furthermore, lifestyle decisions are crucial, encompassing food patterns, exercise routines, and drug consumption. Men's well-being can be impacted by occupational issues such as stress related to the job and exposure to dangerous substances. Socioeconomic position and access to healthcare are examples of social variables that have a major impact. Another essential element is mental health, with men and women experiencing mental health issues such as anxiety and depression in different ways. All things considered, a comprehensive knowledge of men's health necessitates taking into account the complex interactions between these various components.

## THE VALUE OF LEADING A HEALTHY LIFESTYLE

Men must have a healthy lifestyle to reach their highest level of well-being. Frequent exercise is essential because it lowers the risk of chronic illnesses, such as cardiovascular problems, and aids with weight control. Essential nutrients are provided by a diet that is well-balanced and nutrient-rich, promoting general health and avoiding nutritional deficits. Getting enough sleep is equally important for both mental and physical renewal. It is essential to abstain from bad habits like smoking and binge drinking because they are associated with a host of health issues. Managing stress through practices like frequent health check-ups and meditation increases the likelihood of living a long and healthy life. Men can proactively address potential health concerns by adopting a holistic approach to living a healthy lifestyle.

# PREVENTIVE ACTIONS FOR THE HEALTH OF MEN

Men's health is protected and the danger of many diseases is reduced via the use of preventive measures. Frequent check-ups and screenings for health conditions allow for the early identification of possible problems, allowing for prompt intervention. Adherence to vaccination schedules is crucial as vaccinations are a critical component in the prevention of infectious diseases. Frequent physical activity helps avoid diseases like diabetes and obesity in addition to improving general well-being. A heart-healthy diet high in fruits, vegetables, and whole grains can lower the risk of cardiovascular illnesses dramatically. Furthermore, avoiding dangerous behaviors like drug misuse and unprotected sex is essential to preventing STDs and problems from addiction. Men who take proactive steps toward prevention are more equipped to take control of their health and well-being.

# MEN'S HEALTH AND HERBAL MEDICINE

With its origins in customary medicine, herbal therapy has been known for enhancing men's health. It is thought that many herbs have medicinal qualities that can help with a range of health issues. For example, ginseng is popularly used for its energy-boosting and stress-relieving properties, while saw palmetto is frequently utilized to improve prostate health. It is believed that Tribulus terrestris improves the health of male reproduction, and ashwagandha helps manage stress due to its adaptogenic qualities. Herbal medication may or may not be effective, but some men find that these treatments are an excellent addition to traditional medical therapy. To ensure safety and effectiveness, as well as to prevent any potential interactions with prescription medications, herbal medicine must be used cautiously and in consultation with healthcare specialists.

# CHAPTER FOUR

## PLANT-BASED TREATMENTS FOR PROSTATITIS

### OBSERVED PALMETTO

Saw palmetto is a well-known herbal medicine that is frequently used to treat prostatitis, a disorder marked by inflammation of the prostate gland. Saw palmetto, which is derived from the fruit of the Serenoa repens plant, has been used traditionally for many urinary and reproductive conditions in Native American medicine for a very long time. It has become more and more well-liked as a prostatitis treatment, as more people look for complementary and alternative methods to lessen the symptoms of this illness.

### METHOD OF ACTION

Saw palmetto has a complex mode of action when it comes to prostatitis. Fatty acids, one of its main ingredients, are thought to prevent the synthesis of several hormones, notably dihydrotestosterone (DHT).

Prostate gland enlargement, a common cause of prostatitis, is linked to DHT. Saw palmetto may help lessen inflammation and symptoms including pelvic pain and urination issues by regulating hormone levels.

## ADMINISTRATION & DOSAGE

Saw palmetto dosage and administration can differ; therefore people need to speak with healthcare providers for specific guidance. Typically offered as extracts, pills, or capsules, the suggested dosage varies based on symptom intensity and individual reaction, among other things. It is crucial to remember that self-prescribing herbal treatments should be done carefully. To guarantee safety and effectiveness, medical advice should be obtained.

## INVESTIGATIVE RESEARCH

Numerous investigations have examined saw palmetto's possible advantages for prostatitis. Some studies indicate that saw palmetto may provide symptomatic relief for those with chronic prostatitis, while the results are not always definitive. These advantages can include less pelvic pain, better urine flow, and a lower frequency of urination. Nonetheless, the disparities in research designs and participant attributes underscore the want for additional investigation to develop a more conclusive comprehension of saw palmetto's effectiveness in the administration of prostatitis.

## ADVANTAGES OF PROSTATITIS

Saw palmetto's anti-inflammatory qualities are not the only advantages it may have for prostatitis. According to certain research, it might also have antioxidant benefits that improve prostate health in general. Its comparatively low occurrence of adverse effects in contrast to traditional therapies also makes it a desirable choice for people looking for natural solutions.

Saw palmetto is a noteworthy herbal therapy that may be helpful for those who have prostatitis. Its mode of action is the control of hormone levels, specifically the suppression of DHT synthesis. The administration and dosage of medication should be customized to each patient's needs, with a focus on the value of healthcare professionals' advice. Even though studies show encouraging results, more study is necessary to confirm palmetto's status as a trustworthy and successful herbal treatment for prostatitis.

# CHAPTER FIVE

## SCIENTIFIC PROOF

## SQUEAKING NETTLE

Because of its many uses and benefits, stinging nettle, or officially Urtica dioica, is a perennial flowering plant that has been used for generations. The plant is distinguished by its small, hair-like structures and serrated leaves, which produce irritating compounds when touched and provide a stinging sensation. Stinging nettle has drawn interest for its possible medical applications and health advantages despite its initial irritation.

## QUALITIES AND USES

The rich nutrient content is one of stinging nettle's most notable characteristics. The plant is an excellent supplement to conventional medical procedures since it contains vitamins, minerals, and antioxidants. Teas, tinctures, and supplements are frequently made from its leaves. There is a reputation that stinging nettle can help with allergies, arthritis, and bladder problems, among other health disorders.

Stinging nettle has a wide range of uses outside of conventional medicine. Because of its vivid green color, it was once used as a fabric dye. Furthermore, stinging nettle has made its way into the kitchen, where young leaves are prepared as a healthy green vegetable or added to salads. Textiles made from the plant's fibers demonstrate how adaptable this biological resource is.

## RECOMMENDED DOSAGE

The recommended dosage for stinging nettle varies depending on how it is ingested. It's important to follow prescribed dosage instructions whether taking this as a tea, supplement, or in another form to prevent any negative effects. To find the right dosage based on specific health issues and factors, it is best to speak with a healthcare provider.

# MEDICAL RESEARCH

To investigate the stinging nettle's medicinal potential, clinical research has been done. Its anti-inflammatory qualities have been the subject of research to learn more about how it might help in the treatment of inflammatory disorders. Based on preliminary research, stinging nettle may have anti-inflammatory properties, which should be investigated by individuals interested in complementary and alternative medicine.

## ANTI-INFLAMMATORY CHARACTERISTICS

Studies on the effects of stinging nettle on inflammatory diseases including arthritis have been conducted. According to some studies, the plant may help reduce the symptoms of inflammatory joint problems; nevertheless, more studies are required to draw firm findings. There is still much to learn about the mechanisms by which stinging nettle reduces inflammation, which emphasizes the need for more research.

Stinging nettle is a unique plant with a variety of uses, including traditional medical and culinary purposes. Adherence to dosage guidelines is essential, and ongoing clinical research continues to illuminate its putative anti-inflammatory characteristics. As research progresses, a more thorough comprehension of stinging nettle's medicinal advantages can surface, offering insightful information for both conventional and contemporary medical procedures.

# CHAPTER SIX

## ADDITIONAL HERBAL TREATMENTS

## QUERCETIN

Widely found in the plant kingdom, quercetin is a flavonoid that has drawn interest due to its possible medicinal and health effects. Quercetin, which can be found in a variety of fruits, vegetables, and grains, has anti-inflammatory and antioxidant qualities. Its anti-oxidant properties aid in the body's defense against free radicals, lowering oxidative stress and promoting general cellular health. Furthermore, because quercetin may slow down the growth of cancer cells and encourage apoptosis, it has been investigated for possible anti-cancer properties.

## CERNILTON (POLLEN EXTRACT FROM RYE GRASS)

The potential of Cernilton, a natural treatment generated from rye grass pollen, to manage prostate health has been investigated. Cernilton's proponents assert that it might lessen the symptoms of benign prostatic hyperplasia (BPH), an aging-related non-cancerous swelling of the prostate gland. Cernilton may have anti-inflammatory properties and may help with BPH-related urine symptoms, according to certain research. Nevertheless, additional investigation is required to completely comprehend its workings and efficiency.

## EXTRACTS OF POLLEN

Traditional medicine has used pollen extracts, which come from a variety of plant sources, because of their possible health-promoting qualities. These extracts frequently include high concentrations of vitamins, minerals, and bioactive substances that may improve general health. Supplements containing pollen extracts are widely available, and supporters of the product say it can boost vitality, assist the immune system, and increase energy. Although there is some evidence that pollen extracts have nutritional value, it is crucial to remember that there is little scientific study on the specific health advantages of pollen extracts, and further research is required to determine their safety and usefulness.

A variety of herbal medicines with possible health advantages include quercetin, Cernilton (a rye grass pollen extract), and other pollen extracts. Because of its anti-inflammatory and antioxidant qualities, quercetin is being studied in natural medicine. The potential of Cernilton, a protein generated from rye grass pollen, to manage prostate health has been investigated, especially in benign prostatic hyperplasia. Different plant sources of pollen extracts are sold for their nutritional value and possible health advantages, although there is currently little scientific proof of these claims. As with any herbal therapy, it's important to use caution when using these products and seek the counsel of medical specialists for specific recommendations based on unique health situations.

# CHAPTER SEVEN

## DIETARY AND LIFESTYLE SUGGESTIONS

## NUTRITION & DIETARY PLANS FOR HEALTHY PROSTATES

Sustaining a nutritious diet is essential for general health and has a big impact on prostate health. Including a range of fruits and vegetables in one's diet helps support prostate health by providing vital vitamins, minerals, and antioxidants. Particularly advantageous are cruciferous vegetables like broccoli and Brussels sprouts as well as tomatoes, which are high in lycopene. Furthermore, it can be beneficial to include omega-3 fatty acids since they contain anti-inflammatory qualities that may help lower the risk of prostate problems. These can be found in foods like flaxseed and fatty fish.

Red and processed meat consumption should be kept to a minimum because these foods have been linked to a higher risk of prostate issues. It may be better to use lean protein sources such as beans, tofu, and chicken. A balanced diet that includes enough fiber also promotes digestive health and may help to indirectly improve prostate health.

## PHYSICAL ACTIVITY AND EXERCISE

In addition to being essential for cardiovascular health, regular exercise also improves prostate health. Aerobic exercise, including jogging, cycling, or brisk walking, improves general fitness and may lower the chance of prostate problems. Maintaining muscular mass and strength is essential for overall physical well-being and can be achieved through resistance training, which includes bodyweight exercises and weight lifting.

Furthermore, including pelvic floor exercises in a workout regimen can be very beneficial to prostate health. Strengthening the muscles that support the bladder and prostate through exercises like Kegels may help prevent certain problems related to the prostate.

# TECHNIQUES FOR STRESS MANAGEMENT

Prostate health is one area of physical and mental health that might suffer from prolonged stress. To promote general well-being, stress management practices must be put into practice. Activities that promote mental balance and relaxation, like yoga, deep breathing techniques, and mindfulness meditation, can help reduce stress.

Stress management can also involve establishing realistic goals, asking for help from friends, family, or professionals, and keeping a healthy work-life balance. Understanding the link between mental and physical health is crucial because reducing stress can obliquely aid in the prevention of prostate problems.

## SUITABLE SLEEP POSITION

Prostate health is one aspect of general health that depends on getting enough good sleep. Insufficient sleep and irregular sleep patterns have been connected to several health problems, including a higher risk of prostate troubles. Good sleep hygiene includes establishing a regular sleep schedule, making your bedroom comfortable, and avoiding stimulants like caffeine right before bed.

Taking timely action to treat sleep abnormalities, such as sleep apnea, can also help to keep the prostate healthy. The body needs good sleep to heal and replenish, and maintaining good sleep hygiene has advantages for mental and physical health.

## THE EFFECT OF HYDRATION ON PROSTATITIS

In addition to being beneficial for general health, enough hydration can help avoid prostatitis or inflammation of the prostate gland. Maintaining proper hydration facilitates the removal of toxins from the body and promotes the health of the prostate and other organs. People need to remember to drink enough water throughout the day, and they should pay particular attention to how much fluid they consume when engaging in physical activity or warmer areas.

# CHAPTER EIGHT

## INCLUDING HERBAL REMEDIES IN EVERYDAY LIVING

## MAKING HERBAL TEAS AND INFUSIONS

Making herbal infusions and teas is one of the easiest methods to include herbal treatments in daily life. In addition to offering a reassuring and delightful ritual, these preparations enable people to take advantage of the medicinal qualities of different plants. Herbal infusions are made by steeping fresh or dried herbs in hot water to extract their health-promoting properties. Contrarily, teas follow a similar procedure but frequently use a blend of herbs for a more complex flavor. Popular infusions and teas made from herbs include ginger to boost immunity, peppermint to aid with digestion, and chamomile to promote relaxation. By varying the steeping times and experimenting with various combinations, people can customize these mixtures to suit their requirements.

# HOW TO USE HERBS IN COOKING

Herbs have long been used to improve food flavor, but when they are cooked, they also provide health advantages. Herbs like basil, thyme, and rosemary, whether fresh or dried, have a variety of therapeutic uses in addition to enhancing food flavor. For example, turmeric has anti-inflammatory properties, and garlic is believed to strengthen the immune system. People can easily add taste and health to their meals by experimenting with different culinary traditions and using herbs in common recipes.

## HERBAL SUPPLEMENTS: RECOMMENDED DOSES

Supplements offer a simple alternative for individuals looking for a more concentrated dose of herbal medicines. However, it's important to use caution when using herbal supplements and to follow recommended dosage amounts. Comprehending the suggested dosage guarantees that patients obtain the therapeutic advantages without the possibility of unfavorable consequences. To ensure the safe and efficient integration of herbal treatments into everyday routines, speaking with a healthcare expert or herbalist can assist in customizing supplement selections to meet specific health needs.

## POSSIBLE CONTRAINDICATIONS TO CONVENTIONAL MEDICINES

Before incorporating herbal medicines into their daily routine, people should be informed about any possible interactions with prescription drugs. It is important to keep lines of communication open with healthcare practitioners because certain herbs have the potential to interfere with the absorption or effectiveness of certain medications. This is especially important for people who use prescription drugs or manage long-term illnesses. Seeking advice from a medical expert can assist in determining any conflicts and help people make well-informed choices when combining herbal remedies with traditional therapies.

# KEEPING AN EYE ON AND MODIFYING HERBAL REGIMENS

As with any health program, the key to successfully incorporating herbal treatments into daily life is observation and modification. People can adjust their strategy by monitoring their body's reaction to herbal infusions, dietary modifications, or supplements regularly. Herbal regimens should be modified in response to any slight changes in health and well-being, whether they are good or bad. Because each person reacts differently to herbal medicines, flexibility and a customized approach are essential. Consulting with herbalists or medical specialists regularly might yield insightful advice on how to best incorporate herbal treatments into one's lifestyle.

## PROBLEMS AND SOLUTIONS

There are many obstacles to overcome when incorporating herbal therapies into daily life, particularly in a society where modern medicine is frequently prioritized. One major obstacle is the dearth of standardized information and guidelines about herbal medicines, which causes uncertainty for those looking for non-traditional methods of healing. The multiplicity of herbal medicines and the variation in their efficacy across individuals may exacerbate the situation.

The suspicion that those used to conventional care may have of herbal therapies presents another difficulty. For herbal remedies to be widely accepted, extensive research and scientific validation are required to determine their safety and efficacy. Furthermore, to guarantee the responsible incorporation of herbal treatments into everyday health routines, concerns about dose, possible side effects, and interactions with prescription drugs must be carefully considered.

Overcoming these obstacles may include bridging the conventional and current knowledge gaps. A more thorough understanding of herbal medicines can be developed via cooperation between herbalists, traditional healers, and medical specialists. By using an interdisciplinary approach, evidence-based guidelines may be developed, which will make it simpler for people to confidently incorporate herbal medicines into their daily lives.

Addressing issues also requires education at a critical level. Enabling people to make educated decisions regarding herbal therapies requires accurate and easily available information. A more knowledgeable and tolerant society can be created by incorporating herbal education into public health campaigns and mainstream healthcare curricula, promoting a positive coexistence of traditional and contemporary approaches to wellness.

## NEW DEVELOPMENTS IN MEN'S HEALTH

Herbal medicines are becoming more and more popular in the field of men's health as supplemental methods to address particular issues. A growing trend is the use of adaptogenic herbs as a stress management strategy. Stress is a prevalent issue that affects many elements of men's health. The ability of herbs like Rhodiola rosea and ashwagandha to improve stress tolerance and advance general well-being is making them more and more well-liked.

Another area where herbal therapies are becoming more popular is prostate health. For example, some people view palmetto as a natural therapy to support prostate health. Including these herbs in daily routines could have preventive effects, especially when combined with a holistic approach that emphasizes a balanced diet and way of life.

Herbal treatments are also becoming more and more popular as a way to help men's reproductive health and correct hormone imbalances. Researchers are looking into the possibility of using herbs like tribulus terrestris and maca root to help male fertility and hormone balance.

The growing appeal of herbal teas, vitamins, and dietary changes is another indication of the trend in men's health toward more natural and holistic approaches.

This pattern points to a wider recognition of herbal medicines as beneficial elements of a proactive, preventative approach to men's health.

## THE POINT WHERE TRADITIONAL AND MODERN MEDICINE COLLIDE

A special point of interaction between traditional and modern medicine is the use of herbal treatments in everyday living. Traditional medicine offers a plethora of knowledge regarding the therapeutic qualities of numerous plants, much of it derived from centuries-old customs and cultural understanding. In contrast, modern medicine uses scientific rigor and technological breakthroughs to diagnose and cure medical disorders.

Acknowledging each approach's capabilities and utilizing them in concert with one another is the first step toward finding common ground between these two methods. For example, contemporary research can corroborate traditional wisdom and offer a scientific rationale for the effectiveness of herbal medicines. This partnership may result in the creation of standardized herbal formulations that guarantee uniformity in dosage and quality.

A more comprehensive and patient-centered approach is also made possible by the incorporation of herbal treatments into traditional healthcare settings. Acknowledging the value of cultural competence in healthcare, professionals can collaborate with traditional healers to respect the various viewpoints on health and healing by including herbal remedies in treatment programs.

New avenues for integrative and individualized healthcare are made possible by the convergence of traditional and modern medicine. Combining the benefits of both strategies gives people access to a wider range of options for improving their well-being and promotes a more inclusive and all-encompassing approach to health in day-to-day living.